The diagnosis and management of diabetes mellitus

Second Edition

J W Simpson
SDA, BVM&S, MPhil, MRCVS

I

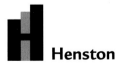

Henston

Henston

*Produced in association with Schering-Plough
Animal Health and Hill's Pet Nutrition*

Henston
A Division of Veterinary Business Development
Olympus House
Werrington Centre
Peterborough PE4 6NA

Telephone: +44 (0)1733 325522
Facsimile: +44 (0) 1733 325512
e-mail: henston@vetsonline.com

Designed and produced by Veterinary Business Development Ltd

ISBN: 1 85054 152 3

Second edition

First published 1994

® 1999 Veterinary Business Development Ltd

Price £7.50

About the author

J W Simpson SDA, BVM&S, MPhil, MRCVS

James Simpson graduated from Edinburgh in 1977 and spent the next three years in mixed practice before returning to the Royal (Dick) School of Veterinary Studies, Edinburgh. In 1983 he obtained an MPhil degree following studies into canine exocrine pancreatic insufficiency.

In 1986 he established and continues to run a gastroenterology referral service at Edinburgh and has published books on gastroenterology and clinical nutrition. He holds a Sir Winston Churchill Fellowship and is an RCVS Specialist in Internal Medicine, Head of Internal Medicine and SeniorLecturer.

III

Contents

IV

List of figures and photographs

V

Preface

The diagnosis and treatment of diabetes mellitus creates a challenging situation for both the pet-owning client and his or her veterinary surgeon. The constant care required, often for most of the pet's life, needs commitment and dedication from the owners as well as considerable time on the part of the veterinary practice to allow a complete explanation of the care and treatment required.

While some owners may be happy to follow instructions without question, the prolonged period of treatment usually means that they will eventually want to know more. Sadly, even the most diligent of veterinary surgeons is unable to devote the large amount of time needed to convey a complete understanding of the condition to concerned owners.

The format of this book is such that it can be read through from cover to cover or, alternatively, referred to as and when required. Reading at their own pace, owners, veterinary students and nurses can obtain a complete understanding of the processes going on inside the diabetic animal and the most appropriate way of managing the condition.

Finally, may I express my sincerest thanks to James Simpson for his hard work and dedication in the production of this book. His authoritative handling of the text and professional approach to the subject, are reflected throughout the volume. Thanks too go to Alison Ridyard* for her assistance with the chapter dealing with feline diabetes mellitus.

David J Watson BVetMed MRCVS

Editor

Alison Ridyard, BVSc, CertSAM, MRCVS, graduated from Bristol University in 1992 and spent the next five years in mixed and small animal practice. In 1998, she took up a residency in Small Animal Internal Medicine at the R(D)SVS, Edinburgh, and gained the RCVS Certificate in Small Animal Medicine.

Introduction

Diabetes mellitus is a common endocrine disorder of the dog and cat. In order to successfully treat the condition, the owner and veterinary surgeon must work closely together. It is obvious, therefore, that an understanding of the disease is essential for both parties if treatment is to be effective.

Although the initial stages of treatment may require the patient to be hospitalised and under veterinary supervision, eventually the owner will have to take over the day to day management of the pet. This is a daunting task for many owners who are often anxious and may feel unable to carry out the procedures necessary for effective management of the condition.

As a consequence, veterinary surgeons will normally spend some time discussing the day to day management with the owner and will usually provide some form of written instructions for the client to keep. Literature produced by drug manufacturers can also be of considerable assistance in providing the necessary information relating to treatment and management.

The purpose of this publication, however, is to offer the practitioner, veterinary undergraduate, veterinary nurse and owner an opportunity to review all the aspects of current knowledge about the condition of diabetes mellitus. It will provide a ready reference for all interested parties and, to help, the information is laid out in distinct sections which should make retrieval of information easier.

To ensure a complete understanding of the disease, we start with information about the incidence of the condition, relevant anatomy and physiology of the gland involved, followed by a discussion of the causes (aetiology), clinical picture, diagnosis and treatment.

In a few rare cases, initial stabilisation of the patient is difficult and occasionally patients who have been stabilised may become unstable. For this reason, a section has been included on how to investigate complications and correct the underlying causes.

It is always dangerous to consider cats as being 'small dogs' when they are a totally individual species developing conditions and exhibiting clinical signs specific to their species. For this reason, a section of the book concentrates on feline diabetes mellitus.

Information is also provided on other conditions of the pancreas, including insulinoma and exocrine pancreatic insufficiency.

This is not a definitive text but a guide which we hope the reader will find of practical value. Additional information is available in the major veterinary medical textbooks for those with a special interest in endocrine disorders.

Medical terminology is used throughout the text and the lay reader is encouraged to use the extensive glossary to gain a better understanding of these terms.

1 Incidence of diabetes mellitus

Diabetes mellitus is one of the most common endocrine conditions seen in dogs. The condition occurs in approximately one in every 200 middle-aged dogs and is especially common in the smaller breeds such as Poodles, Terriers and Dachshunds. This does not preclude the condition occurring in large breeds especially Cocker Spaniels, German Shepherds, Boxers, Samoyeds and Rottweilers. A genetic predisposition has been suggested in the Keeshund, Cairn Terrier and Miniature Pinscher.

Diabetes mellitus is seen most frequently in middle-aged dogs, usually between the ages of seven and nine years. The majority of cases occur in entire females (66%) due to the influence of the reproductive hormones (see later). Neutered females and males are less commonly affected. Diabetes mellitus occasionally occurs in immature dogs of either sex.

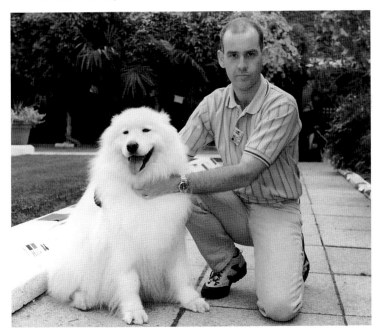

Figure 1.
Diabetic dogs, with suitable treatment, can lead normal lives.
(Courtesy of Hill's Pet Nutrition).

2 Anatomy and physiology of the pancreas

The pancreas is a pink, lobulated V-shaped gland which lies in close association with the stomach and the duodenum in the cranial abdomen (Figure 2). The gland is composed of exocrine and endocrine cells. The exocrine cells account for more than 90% of the total pancreas and produce digestive enzymes which drain into the duodenum via the pancreatic ducts *(Appendix 3 discusses exocrine pancreatic disorders)*. The endocrine pancreas is composed of small islands of cells called the Islets of Langerhans, which are scattered throughout the exocrine tissue.

There are four types of cell in the Islets of Langerhans: alpha cells which secrete glucagon, beta cells which secrete insulin, delta cells which secrete somatostatin and F cells which secrete pancreatic polypeptide. The alpha cells are found in greatest concentration round the periphery of the Islets while beta cells are concentrated in the centre.

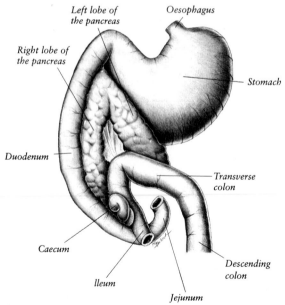

Figure 2.
Location of the pancreas in relation to the stomach and duodenum in the dog.
(Courtesy of Hill's Atlas of Veterinary Clinical Anatomy).

Both glucagon and insulin are polypeptide hormones responsible for maintaining blood glucose levels. In more general terms, these hormones influence carbohydrate, protein and fat metabolism. The ability to maintain blood glucose levels within fine limits (4 to 5.5mmol/l) is due to the antagonistic (or opposing) action of these two hormones as shown in Figure 3.

	Insulin	Glucagon
Secretion causes	Decrease in blood glucose	Increase in blood glucose
Secretion stimulated by	Increase in blood glucose	Decrease in blood glucose
Secretion also stimulated by	–	Release of insulin
Uptake of glucose by peripheral cells	Increased	–
Protein breakdown	Inhibited	–
Fat breakdown	Inhibited	–
Glycogen breakdown	Inhibited	Stimulated
Gluconeogenesis	Inhibited	Stimulated
Formation of glycogen	Stimulated	–

Figure 3.
A description of the antagonistic effects of insulin and glucagon on protein, carbohydrate and fat metabolism.

3 Classification of diabetes mellitus

Diabetes mellitus is associated with a relative or absolute lack of insulin which in turn results in a disturbance of carbohydrate, fat and protein metabolism. The classification of diabetes mellitus in dogs and cats is similar to that used in man, being based on the pathophysiology and pathogenic effects on beta cells. Cases of diabetes mellitus may be divided into the following two types:

Type I

This represents the most common form of diabetes mellitus in dogs. Affected animals have a high resting blood glucose level, low resting insulin level and fail to secrete insulin in the presence of developing hyperglycaemia. These dogs have insulin dependent diabetes mellitus associated with a total loss of functional beta cells. In some cases there may be a gradual loss of insulin secretion as the beta cells are destroyed.

They may be initially controlled with oral hypoglycaemic drugs and dietary management but ultimately they become insulin dependent. Causes of this total loss of beta cells and Type I disease include: immune mediated disease, genetic predisposition, pancreatitis and prolonged exposure to insulin antagonist hormones (phaeochromocytoma).

Type II

This type of diabetes mellitus is characterised by insulin resistance rather than a loss of beta cells. Affected dogs have a high resting blood glucose level and a normal or high resting insulin level. Although the insulin level varies, beta cells fail to respond to increasing blood glucose by secreting more insulin. These dogs may initially be non insulin dependent but ultimately become Type I insulin dependent diabetics.

Resistance to or inhibition of insulin secretion may occur as a result of overeating and obesity, elevated levels of growth hormone or the administration of glucocorticoids and thyroxine. As a consequence of insulin resistance, beta cells increase output of insulin, hence the normal or high circulating insulin levels observed in Type II diabetes. Type I disease only occurs if resistance persists and beta cells become completely exhausted.

Attempts have previously been made to differentiate between insulin dependent diabetes and non insulin dependent diabetes in dogs. This involved the use of various secretagogue tests including the intravenous glucose tolerance test and the intravenous glucagon tolerance test, but results have been inconsistent and unreliable. For these reasons the tests are no longer used and the clinical decision to use insulin therapy should be based on the severity of the clinical signs exhibited by the patient.

In early cases, where the patient remains bright, active, shows no weight loss and has no signs of ketoacidosis, oral hypoglycaemic drugs and dietary management may be tried. Where these serious and advanced clinical signs are present, insulin therapy must be used immediately.

4 Aetiology

Diabetes mellitus may be described as an endocrine disorder which results in interference with protein, fat and carbohydrate metabolism. This effect on metabolism is brought about by either a relative or absolute deficiency in insulin. This, as might be expected, is an over-simplification of the situation as other factors play an important role in the aetiology of diabetes mellitus (Figure 4).

In normal animals, the response to raised blood glucose (hyperglycaemia) is an increase in circulating insulin which in turn stimulates the insulin receptors on peripheral tissue cells to permit movement of glucose into the cells. Other actions are described in Figure 3. As the glucose is taken up by peripheral cells, the blood glucose level falls and this changes the balance between circulating insulin and glucagon. Glucagon now predominates and increases the blood glucose level by reducing cellular uptake by cells and stimulates glycogenolysis and gluconeogenesis.

In diabetes mellitus the inability to produce insulin results in a failure of glucose uptake by peripheral cells, leading to hyperglycaemia, and failure of the other insulin dependent processes shown in Figure 3. As a result, the normal balance between circulating insulin and glucagon levels is lost. Levels of glucagon which would normally be depressed by increasing blood glucose may remain, stimulating glycogenolysis and gluconeogenesis in the liver. As the cells are effectively 'starved' of glucose and therefore energy, alternative sources of fuel are utilised. There is an increase in protein breakdown with amino acids being used for gluconeogenesis. Fat breakdown to fatty acids proceeds faster than normal oxidation pathways can handle. Consequently, acetone and beta hydroxybutyric acid, normally absent, are produced and accumulate in the circulation, resulting in the characteristic 'ketotic' smell on the breath of diabetics. These fatty acids also induce a metabolic acidosis and are toxic to the central nervous system, resulting in signs of depression, anorexia and vomiting associated with the condition ketoacidosis.

Both fat and protein catabolism result in weight loss. Hyperglycaemia gives rise to a loss of glucose in the urine (glycosuria) once the renal threshold for glucose (10 to 12mmol/l) is reached. The high level of glucose in the urine induces a loss of water from the body (osmotic diuresis) leading to polyuria and compensatory polydipsia. The satiety and feeding centres located in the hypothalamus of the brain are also affected by falling insulin levels. Glucose entering the cells of the satiety centre normally reduces the desire to eat and gives a feeling of feeding satisfaction. However, movement of glucose into these cells is dependent on insulin so that in diabetes mellitus, glucose is unable to enter the cells in spite of the hyperglycaemia, satiety does not occur and the animal remains hungry (polyphagia).

Therefore, the classical signs of diabetes mellitus, polyuria, polydipsia, polyphagia and weight loss can all be explained.

Some of the other agents shown in Figure 4 may contribute to the aetiology in the following manner:

- Pancreatic Hypoplasia

- Obesity

- Immune mediated disease

- Hormonal antagonism   *Growth hormone*
                             Glucocorticoids
                             Progestogens
                             Progesterone
                             Hyperadrenocorticalism
                             Glucagon

- Pancreatitis.

- Phaeochromocytoma

Figure 4.
Factors which are implicated in the aetiology of canine diabetes mellitus.

Obesity

Obesity occurs when there is an excessive intake of energy over expenditure. The excess energy cannot be immediately utilised by the body and is therefore converted to fat and stored as adipose tissue.

Many diabetic dogs are obese and there is evidence to suggest that obese dogs are hyperinsulinaemic and may be insulin resistant, that is the insulin does not produce the expected effects. Insulin resistance may be due to loss of insulin receptor sites, reduced insulin receptor sensitivity or to other defects in cell function. Loss of insulin receptor sites may be due to the development of hyperglycaemia associated with overeating.

There appears to be a direct correlation between the degree of obesity and level of insulin resistance. Ultimately, the effects of relative insulin deficiency (post receptor defects) occur, exacerbating the inability of glucose to enter peripheral cells, thus leading to Type II diabetes.

Progesterone

Diabetes mellitus is more commonly observed in entire females than in neutered females or males. Bitches may develop transient diabetes during oestrus or pregnancy due to the antagonistic actions of progesterone. These symptoms may resolve once anoestrus occurs or following parturition. Such bitches, however, are highly likely to develop Type I diabetes mellitus at a subsequent oestrus.

Production of growth hormone is stimulated during dioestrus or following the administration of certain progestogens or progesterone. Growth hormone is diabetogenic and appears to induce insulin receptor resistance and consequently hyperglycaemia and hyperinsulinaemia, the hallmarks of Type II diabetes.

As the influence of growth hormone is maintained, beta cell exhaustion occurs and circulating levels of insulin fall. Removal of progesterone is important in the long-term management of diabetes mellitus, reducing the diabetogenic effects of growth hormone. This is why it is recommended to neuter females following the diagnosis of diabetes mellitus.

Glucocorticoids

Patients receiving long-term administration of glucocorticoids or those with hyperadrenocorticalism may develop diabetes mellitus.

Glucocorticoids are diabetogenic and interfere with insulin receptors on peripheral tissue cells, preventing glucose uptake by the cells. Hyperinsulinaemia develops in an attempt to force glucose into the cells and if glucocorticoid administration persists, overt diabetes mellitus may develop as a result of beta cell exhaustion.

Pancreatitis

Both acute and chronic pancreatitis are relatively common in the dog. Although diabetes mellitus associated with pancreatitis is reported in the literature, it is rare. Significant on-going inflammation leading to destruction of both exocrine and endocrine cells is required before overt diabetes is likely to occur. In spite of such damage, exocrine pancreatic dysfunction is far more likely than diabetes in the dog.

Immune mediated disease

In man, immune mediated disease is an important factor in the development of diabetes mellitus and this may be true for the dog as well. Immune mediated insulitis, anti beta cells antibodies and auto antibodies have been reported in the dog. For this immune mediated mechanism to activate, many factors must be satisfied. The dog must be genetically predisposed to diabetes and environmental factors such as the administration of drugs or exposure to infective agents is required to trigger development of antibody against beta cells.

Once satisfied, there is a slow progressive loss of beta cells which will remain sub-clinical in the early stages but will eventually result in the development of typical symptoms associated with diabetes mellitus.

9

Phaeochromocytoma

Tumours of the adrenal medulla produce excessive amounts of catacholamines such as adrenaline and noradrenaline. These hormones have an inhibitory effect on insulin production which results in very low circulating insulin levels and predisposes to diabetes mellitus.

5 History and clinical signs

Clinically, diabetes mellitus can be divided into two forms:

- Those animals which are generally bright but display polyphagia, polyuria and polydipsia. Obesity or some degree of weight loss may have been noted.

- Those animals which are ketoacidotic and present with depression, anorexia, vomiting and dehydration.

In the entire bitch, clinical signs are often observed following a recent oestrus and the history may suggest episodes of polyuria and polydipsia associated with previous oestrous cycles. Although the dog will lose weight with diabetes, they initially may be obese. Blindness may occur associated with the development of cataracts and is seen in 25% of cases. Enlargement of the liver (hepatomegaly) may be detected in 50% of cases.

Most early cases present as bright, alert dogs with a history of sudden or gradual onset of polyuria and polydipsia. The extent of the PUPD will vary but usually dogs will drink in excess of 100ml/kg/day. Weight loss will also occur in spite of a ravenous appetite.

As the condition progresses, the clinical picture changes. The initial signs of polyphagia, polyuria and polydipsia will be superseded as the patient develops ketoacidosis and becomes depressed, anorexic, vomits and exhibits dehydration. The breath may have a sweet smell of acetone. The development of ketoacidosis should be viewed as a serious progression of the disease and if left untreated will lead to diabetic coma and death.

6 Differential diagnosis

Although clinical signs such as PUPD and polyphagia, weight loss and ketotic breath strongly suggest diabetes mellitus, not all these signs are present in every clinical case and may be observed in other clinical conditions. The differential diagnosis, or other conditions which may be confused with diabetes mellitus, are as follows:

- Diabetes insipidus
- Chronic renal failure
- Hyperadrenocorticalism
- Psychogenic polydipsia
- Pyometra
- Hepatic disease
- Fanconi syndrome
- Post prandial hyperglycaemia
- Drugs effect; steroids, progestogens
- Intravenous glucose infusion
- Laboratory error
- Oestrus
- Stress (especially in the cat)

Figure 5.
The differential diagnosis which should be considered when dogs are presented with hyperglycaemia, polyuria and or polydipsia.

Diabetes insipidus (DI)

The dog's ability to concentrate its urine and conserve water is largely controlled by antidiuretic hormone (ADH) which is produced by the pituitary gland when the body needs to conserve water. The hormone acts on the collecting ducts of the kidney tubules and gives rise to water resorption and thus concentration of the urine.

If the pituitary gland fails to produce ADH or the collecting ducts fail to respond to the hormone, the urine will remain dilute and significant water loss from the body will occur. The only way water balance can now be restored is by increasing water intake. In spite of drinking excessively, dogs never manage to regain water balance and become dehydrated. Dogs with DI generally drink considerably more than those with diabetes mellitus, always exceeding 100ml/kg/day, and produce consistently dilute urine with a specific gravity of 1.000 to 1.009. Urinalysis will reveal no evidence of protein, blood, ketones, glucose or significant deposit. There will be no response to the partial water deprivation test although most cases will respond to the ADH test.

The partial water deprivation test confirms the dog is unable to concentrate its urine due either to failure in ADH production or to collecting duct dysfunction. The ADH test is used to confirm a significant lack of ADH production by the pituitary gland. Following an injection of ADH, an immediate increase in urine concentration will be observed if the problem is the result of a pituitary gland defect. If the problem is associated with the collecting ducts failing to respond to ADH or there is renal medullary washout present, no increase in urine concentration will occur. These tests must be carried out under strict veterinary supervision as the patient can rapidly become dehydrated.

Psychogenic polydipsia (PP)

This condition is very difficult to differentiate from DI as the clinical and diagnostic features are very similar. In PP, however, there is usually no response to either the partial water deprivation test or the ADH test because the problem is associated with medullary washout and not the collecting ducts. Frequently, PP is associated with stress or boredom and cases will respond to a change in routine and to partial water deprivation carried out under veterinary supervision.

Hyperadrenocorticalism (HAC)

The adrenal glands can be found just in front of each kidney. The gland is divided into the cortex, which produces a hormone called cortisol responsible for many metabolic functions, and the medulla which produces adrenaline and noradrenaline. The pituitary gland produces a hormone called adrenocorticotrophic hormone (ACTH) which stimulates the adrenal cortex to produce cortisol in times of need.

In HAC, an excessive production of cortisol occurs leading to diverse clinical signs, many of which are common to diabetes mellitus. In addition to these, dogs with HAC often exhibit an enlarged pendulous abdomen, bilateral symmetrical alopecia of the flanks, muscle weakness, hepatomegaly and calcinosis cutis.

Although hyperglycaemia and hyperinsulinaemia are common in HAC, only some 8% of cases will have or develop diabetes mellitus. The blood glucose level is usually only moderately elevated (8 to 10mmol/l) and so glycosuria is not consistently present. Changes in the blood picture include leucocytosis, neutrophilia, lymphopaenia, and eosinopaenia as well as an increase in serum alkaline phosphatase.

Response to the administration of ACTH together with the low and high dose dexamethasone tests can be used to confirm the diagnosis. In addition, it is now possible to measure serum ACTH levels which can help to determine the type of HAC present. These are complex tests which require careful interpretation which is outside the scope of this publication. The reader is referred to a veterinary medical textbook for further information.

Chronic renal failure (CRF)

The kidneys contain many thousands of nephrons which are responsible for filtering the blood and removing waste products into the urine. Dogs have more nephrons than they require for normal health; however, any which are damaged are not replaced and thus the total number of nephrons declines throughout life. Chronic renal failure occurs when the nephrons have been reduced until inadequate numbers remain to maintain normal kidney function (<25%).

Most dogs with CRF are polyuric and polydipsic and may also display an increase in waste products in the blood (azotaemia). Blood urea and creatinine are two of the most commonly measured waste products in CRF. If the blood urea and creatinine levels in the circulation become high, the dog may become depressed, anorexic, start to vomit and subsequently become dehydrated. Urine is often isothenuric and may contain evidence of protein, blood, granular casts and inflammatory cells.

Pyometra

Pyometra usually occurs shortly after oestrus or following the frequent use of progestagen therapy to control breeding. Polyuria and polydipsia may be the predominant clinical signs but glycosuria does not occur in this condition. The presence of a vaginal discharge depends on whether the cervix is open or closed and is an inconsistent finding. Abdominal enlargement may occur in the closed form of the condition.

Most patients with pyometra become toxic and exhibit signs of depression, anorexia, vomiting and dehydration. There is usually an increase in the number of circulating white blood cells (leucocytosis) and evidence of azotaemia.

Liver disease

The clinical signs associated with liver disease are mostly non specific but may include polyuria and polydipsia. Depending on the type and severity of the liver disease present, dogs may be hypoglycaemic or hyperglycaemic, making the clinical picture similar to diabetes mellitus. Where liver disease is suspected, liver enzyme and function tests should be carried out together with urinalysis, which may sometimes reveal the presence of biurate crystals. A definitive diagnosis normally requires the collection of a liver biopsy for histopathological examination.

Fanconi syndrome

Fanconi syndrome is associated with a primary defect in the renal tubular absorptive function which may be inherited or acquired, following heavy metal poisoning. Clinically, dogs exhibit PUPD and diagnostically the condition is characterised by glycosuria without accompanying hyperglycaemia. In addition to the glycosuria, there are also significant losses of amino acids, phosphate and other important electrolytes.

7 Diagnosis

The diagnosis of diabetes mellitus is based on:

- Confirmation of the presence of PUPD by measuring water intake over a 24-hour period. Classically, dogs with diabetes mellitus will drink in excess of 80ml/kg/day and often 100ml/kg/day.

- Urinalysis will reveal glycosuria (>2%) and the urine specific gravity will usually be normal in spite of the PUPD, due to the presence of large amounts of glucose. Secondary urinary tract infection is common in diabetic patients.

- A persistently elevated fasting blood glucose level above the renal threshold of 10 to 12mmol/l.

- The documentation of concurrent ketonuria and a sweet smell on the breath confirms the presence of ketoacidosis.

- Serum fructosamine levels are usually elevated, confirming the loss of glycaemic control over the preceding three weeks. Although not used routinely for the diagnosis of diabetes mellitus in the dog, it can be of considerable value in the cat where stress hyperglycaemia makes the diagnosis of diabetes mellitus difficult.

- Although non specific for diabetes mellitus, serum biochemistry will often reveal an elevation in serum alanine aminotransferase, alkaline phosphatase, triglycerides and cholesterol. In ketoacidosis there may be elevations in blood urea and creatinine and decreased sodium (hyponatraemia) and potassium (hypokalaemia) levels.

15

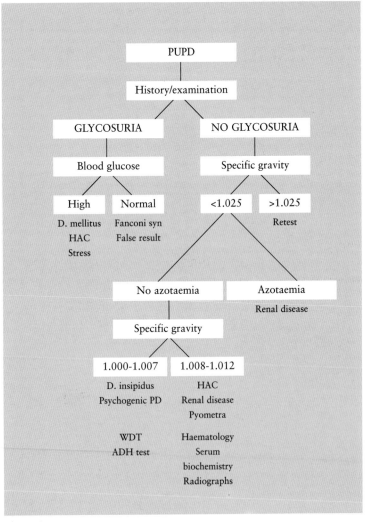

Figure 6.
Algorithm for the investigation of polyuria (PU) and polydipsia (PD) in dogs.

8 Therapy

The aims of therapy may be summarised as follows:

- Correct ketoacidosis and dehydration if present.

- Remove any underlying cause or predisposing factor. In particular, entire females should be spayed once they are stabilised and all progestagen and corticosteroid therapy stopped if it is safe to do so. Treatment for concurrent hyperadrenocorticalism should be initiated if appropriate.

- Restoration of blood glucose levels to as near normal as possible. This will reduce the risk of long-term complications such as cataract, neuropathy and nephropathy.

- Correct glycosuria, so reversing the PUPD.

- Correct any concurrent cystitis using an appropriate antibiotic.

- Restore normal body weight if the patient is either under weight or obese.

Therapy for diabetes mellitus normally requires a combination of insulin administration and strict dietary management. It is extremely unusual for canine diabetes to respond to oral hypoglycaemic drugs. The following section describes the different components of therapy in more detail.

Dietary management

Dietary management plays an essential role in the treatment of diabetes mellitus. Its aim is to provide a balanced diet, reduce post-prandial glucose fluctuations and correct either cachexia or obesity. It is important to ensure the main meal coincides with peak circulating insulin levels.

Types of diet

A diet for most obese diabetics should contain a high level of fibre and complex carbohydrates such as starch, rather than simple monosaccharides and disaccharides which cause marked fluctuations in blood glucose level (see under stabilisation). For these reasons, a tinned or dry commercial diet designed for diabetics should be used rather than a semi-moist diet.

Dietary composition

Currently, the fat content of the diet is recommended to be no more than 15% dry matter (DM) because dogs with diabetes already have altered lipid metabolism which could be further compromised. The majority of calories should be provided by complex carbohydrate (50 to 55% DM).

Dietary fibre is primarily composed of polysaccharide which cannot be digested and so remains within the intestinal lumen and passes out in the faeces. Fibre can be classified into soluble (gums and pectins) and insoluble fibre (cellulose) each having different properties. The beneficial effect of fibre in canine diabetics is not affected by the type of fibre fed. Dietary fibre is beneficial in the treatment of diabetics for several reasons:

- It can be used to reduce the calorie content of the diet and so control obesity.

- It slows down the rate of carbohydrate absorption from the intestine.

- It reduces the post-prandial fluctuations in blood glucose levels; this in turn reduces glycosuria and the patient's insulin requirement.

- Ideally, the diet should contain between 13 and 18% DM fibre. However, care is required when using very high fibre diets as very high fibre may lead to poor palatability. As it is essential for diabetic animals to eat regular meals, poor palatability will affect stabilisation.

Protein should be of high biological value (quality) and constitute some 20 to 25% DM of the diet. This level and quality of protein should ensure it is used efficiently for restoring tissue protein and not simply as an energy source. A lower level of protein may be required where there is concurrent nephropathy present.

Many dogs with diabetes mellitus are obese. Correction of the obesity should be an important part of the treatment regime as it improves the responsiveness of peripheral tissues to insulin and reduces hyperglycaemia. Middle-aged dogs should normally receive 40-60kcal/kg/day calculated on their ideal body weight. Obese dogs should receive a high fibre commercial low calorie diet in order to restore ideal body weight, such as described above.

Where the dog is initially under weight, it is desirable to restore body weight to normal using an energy dense, highly digestible diet before placing the animal on a high fibre diet.

Obtaining the correct balance of protein, carbohydrate, fat and fibre using home-made diets is difficult to achieve and even more difficult to maintain on a day to day basis. For this reason, a commercial veterinary diet should be fed in preference to home-made diets (see Figure 7).

In addition, owners must be extremely careful to ensure that dogs receive *no* additional sources of food. Variations in the amount of food given each day and timing of meals can seriously interfere with stabilisation (see stabilisation).

Hill's* Prescription Diet* Canine w/d*: for dogs of normal body weight.

Hill's* Prescription Diet* Canine r/d*: for obese dogs.

Hill's* Prescription Diet* Canine i/d*: for under weight dogs.

Figure 7.
Diets which have been specially formulated for the dietary management of canine diabetes mellitus.

Water

In all cases, diabetics should have free access to a supply of fresh, clean water at all times. Other than the practical inconvenience, polyuria and polydipsia have no detrimental effect on the patient's well-being.

Feeding schedule

Feeding schedules should be designed to enhance the effectiveness of injected insulin and reduce the post-prandial fluctuations in blood glucose. The best results will be obtained if one of the following feeding regimes is used:

- Feed one quarter of the daily ration followed by the daily insulin injection first thing in the morning. The remaining three-quarters of the daily ration should be fed eight hours later to coincide with the peak insulin activity.

- Some dogs benefit from twice daily insulin injections. In this regime the dog should be fed half of its daily ration first thing in the morning followed by its insulin injection. The remaining half ration should be fed 12 hours later with the second insulin injection.

Exercise

Exercise has an important part to play in helping to maintain glycaemic control. It helps to promote weight loss and will help to reverse insulin resistance which is caused by obesity. It also lowers blood glucose levels by increasing blood flow to the site of insulin injection and stimulating insulin mobilisation. Although diabetics should be encouraged to take regular exercise, it is important that significant day to day variations in the amount and timing of exercise are avoided.

Hypoglycaemic drugs

Although oral hypoglycaemic drugs are available for the treatment of diabetes in man, they are rarely effective in the dog as most of these patients are insulin dependent. Oral hypoglycaemic drugs, however, may be of value in the cat (see later).

There are two classes of hypoglycaemic drug available:

- The sulphonylureas, which act by stimulating beta cell secretion and therefore depend on the presence of some functional beta cells. They also increase the sensitivity of peripheral insulin receptors and so increase glucose uptake by cells. However, sulphonylureas may be detrimental to liver function.

- The biguanides: the mode of action of biguanides such as metformin is not fully understood but may involve increasing peripheral cell utilisation of glucose, increasing insulin receptor binding and inhibition of hepatic glucose production.

Dose regimes for these drugs are shown in Figure 8.

Group	Drug (trade name)	Dose
Biguanides	Metformin (Glucophage)	250 to 500mg tid
Sulphonylureas	Glipizide (Glibenese)	0.25 to 0.5mg/kg bid
	Chlorpropamide (Diabinese)	10 to 40mg/kg divided

Figure 8.
Some hypoglycaemic drugs which may be used in the treatment of canine diabetes mellitus. It is important to note that these drugs are not licensed for veterinary use.

Insulin

The majority of diabetic dogs are insulin dependent and require daily injections of insulin together with strict dietary management to maintain stability. There are large numbers of human insulin products available but only two pharmaceutical companies produce veterinary licensed products (Figure 9). In general, insulins may be classified according to their composition.

Trade name	Species	Strength	Route	Peak	Duration
INSUVET for dog/cat					
Neutral	Bovine	100iu/ml	I/v or I/m	1-1½ hours	2 hours
Lente	Bovine	100iu/ml	S/c	6-12 hours	24 hours
Protamine Zinc	Bovine	100iu/ml	S/c	12-24 hours	36 hours
CANINSULIN for dogs					
Mixed	Porcine	40iu/ml	S/c	3-12 hours	8-24 hours

Figure 9.
Types of veterinary insulin which are available, giving details of their composition, strength and duration of activity.

Neutral insulin

These are also known as soluble insulins and are the *only* form of insulin which can be used intravenously or intramuscularly. They are primarily used in the treatment of ketoacidosis because they have a very rapid onset of action but short duration of activity (two hours) allowing good therapeutic control.

Lente insulin

These insulins are designed for use in the long-term management of diabetes and *must* be given by subcutaneous injection. They are intermediate in action, having their peak effect about eight hours after injection and lasting for about 24 hours. There are obvious advantages to using insulin with a 24-hour duration of activity.

Protamine Zinc insulin

This is a long-acting insulin which may be used in the long-term management of diabetes by subcutaneous injection. This produces its peak effect eight to 12 hours after administration and lasts for up to 36 hours. Where patients rapidly metabolise insulin, these long-acting types may provide better control, lasting for the ideal 24 hours rather than 36 hours.

Mixed insulins

One of the veterinary insulins is supplied as a mixture of amorphous zinc insulin and crystalline zinc insulin. By mixing the different types of insulin it is possible to alter the duration of circulating insulin levels. Amorphous insulin gives a peak effect at three hours after injection and lasts some eight hours while the other insulin works more slowly with a peak effect at eight to 12 hours and gradually declines within 24 hours.

Species insulins

Bovine and porcine insulin are derived from the pancreas of the respective species while human insulin is produced by recombinant DNA technology. There is no specific canine insulin available commercially but porcine insulin is identical to naturally occurring canine insulin and rarely results in an immune response, i.e. antibody production in response to injected foreign protein. Beef and human insulins differ in structure from canine insulin by one or two amino acids and on rare occasions have been known to induce an immune response in dogs. Despite this, beef insulin is better in the treatment of diabetic dogs because blood levels tail off more slowly and so do not normally allow the abrupt decline observed with porcine insulin. It is also preferable in dogs which have antibodies to their own insulin.

Strengths of insulin

All insulins used in man and most veterinary insulins have been standardised to 100iu/ml, although one veterinary insulin is available at the lower concentration of 40iu/ml.

Sterile, disposable, graduated syringes are used to administer insulin with the graduations marked on the syringe making loading of insulin easier for the client and ensuring accuracy. Care must be taken to ensure the correct type of syringe is used with the correct veterinary insulin. The 100iu/ml syringes have the graduations marked in black while the 40iu/ml syringes have graduations marked in red.

Treatment of the uncomplicated case

Where the dog is PUPD, polyphagic but bright and alert without signs of ketoacidosis, it is described as having uncomplicated diabetes. Those patients which have been successfully treated for their ketoacidosis and are now eating may also be considered uncomplicated cases. In both situations, the treatment regimes described below may be initiated.

They usually respond well to establishing a good daily routine which involves regular measurement of either urine glucose or blood glucose in conjunction with insulin injections and dietary management. The two regimes are described below.

(i) Stabilisation using urine glucose measurements

Although measurement of urine glucose is not ideal and is now losing favour in veterinary medicine, it can be a very successful method of stabilising some dogs. It is a simple and easy way for the client to monitor glycaemic control. However, the ease by which blood glucose can now be measured and the availability of fructosamines in assessing glycaemic control have made this method less accurate in the long term.

For this method of stabilisation, patients should ideally be hospitalised, although this is not essential. In any case, careful records should be kept every day throughout the stabilisation period. The daily routine for stabilisation using urine glucose estimations should be as follows:

- 8am: collect urine sample and measure urine glucose level with Keto-diastix. Record the value together with the presence of any ketones in the urine.

- Feed the dog one quarter of its daily ration.

- Calculate the daily insulin dose. On the first day give 0.5iu/kg lente insulin subcutaneously. This should only be given if the dog eats its first meal of the day. On subsequent days the dose of insulin required can be determined from the urine glucose estimation using the following table.

Urine Glucose		Dose
%	mmol/l	
1 to 2	56 - 111	Previous day's dose + 2iu
1/2	28	Previous day's dose + 1iu
1/4	14	Previous day's dose.
0	0	Previous day's dose - 2iu

- Eight hours after the first meal the remaining three-quarters of the daily ration should be fed.

- If hypoglycaemia is going to occur, then it is most likely just prior to feeding the main meal of the day. A careful watch for signs of hypoglycaemia should be made during this time. If signs do occur, the timing of the main meal should be brought forward as it indicates the peak insulin effect is occurring before the main meal is fed.

Initial stabilisation as described above may take two weeks to achieve. During this time the amount of insulin injected will increase each day before settling out at a steady figure. The urine glucose should be just positive each morning and there should be no signs of ketonuria.

Instruction to owners

At this time the hospitalised patient may be sent home with detailed instructions (see Appendix 1), together with a supply of insulin, syringes, Keto-diastix and a suitable veterinary diet. Several commercial companies produce excellent leaflets on diabetes which provide additional information for the owner.

Owners should keep a careful note of daily urine glucose values, presence of ketonuria and the amount of insulin injected. If owners observe the presence of ketones in the urine, they should be instructed to seek veterinary advice immediately, as this is likely to indicate instability. Where an entire female has become diabetic, she should be spayed at the earliest opportunity and certainly before her next oestrus.

If the injection of insulin is carried out incorrectly by the owner, he or she should not repeat the injection as this may lead to insulin over-dosage and hypoglycaemia. In this situation, simply record the error and continue the normal daily routine.

If the dog fails to eat its first meal of the day, only half the insulin dose should be injected. A note should be made on the daily record card and the dog observed for signs of hypoglycaemia. Attempts should be made to encourage the dog to eat at its next scheduled meal.

Owners should be aware of the clinical signs associated with hypoglycaemia. Initially, dogs will become depressed and exhibit muscle tremors, weakness and ataxia. These signs will be followed rapidly by collapse and diabetic coma. Early recognition is important and owners should administer orally a glucose-rich solution such as honey or sugar. Oral glucose should not be administered to patients which are collapsed or unconscious. In such circumstances they should take the dog to the veterinary surgeon as quickly as possible where an intravenous infusion will be administered.

RECORDING CHART

Patient's name: _____
Owner's name & address: _____

INSUVET

Type of insulin: _____
Time(s) of injection: _____ Type of food: _____
Times of feeding: _____

Date	Time of urine collection	Results of urine analysis	Time of Insuvet injection	Units of Insuvet given	Time of feeding a.m.	p.m.	Amount of food (g) a.m.	p.m.	Daily water intake (ml)	Weight (kg)	Additional observations

PRESENTED WITH
THE COMPLIMENTS OF
SCHERING-PLOUGH
ANIMAL HEALTH

Schering-Plough Animal Health

INSUVET

Figure 10.
The table shows how a record can be kept of the dog's daily routine. The photograph shows a specific dog tag which can be worn by a diabetic dog and will warn anyone finding the dog that it requires insulin daily.
(Courtesy of Schering-Plough Animal Health).

(ii) Stabilisation using blood glucose measurement

It is now more common for diabetic patients to be stabilised using blood glucose rather than urine glucose estimations. In the former case, a supply of Glucostix and a glucometer are required. This allows blood glucose measurements to be made using very small amounts of fresh blood.

The daily regime should be as follows:

- Feed a quarter of the daily ration first thing in the morning.

- Then inject the calculated daily insulin, on the first occasion using 0.5iu/kg lente insulin subcutaneously.

- Blood glucose levels should be measured at the time of injection – 11am, 3pm and 5pm on the first day.

- The main meal of the day should be fed eight hours after the insulin injection to coincide with peak insulin activity.

- As it can take the diabetic patient several days to equilibrate to the changes following insulin administration, maintain the same dose for at least three days before repeating the blood glucose estimations at the times given above. The dose of insulin can then be adjusted according to the values recorded.

Twice daily insulin injections

Some patients will respond well to once daily insulin injections; however, many other patients benefit from dividing the dose of insulin into two equal parts given 12 hours apart. In these cases, the diet should be split into two equal parts and given prior to each injection.

Patient monitoring

Monitoring the patient's response to treatment will help to ensure good glycaemic control is maintained and complications are reduced to a minimum. Once initial stabilisation is successfully completed, regular three-weekly check-ups should be established. They should assess the following:

- Observe the patient for recurrence of clinical signs.

- Assess the patient's body weight, adjust diet accordingly.

- Carry out serial blood glucose estimations over one day, and adjust insulin accordingly.

- Measure serum fructosamine levels. Fructosamines are serum proteins which have undergone non enzymatic binding with glucose. The degree of binding is dependent on the amount of glucose present in the circulation and the life-span of the protein (usually three weeks). This is a very useful indicator of glycaemic control over the preceding three weeks and may eliminate the need for serial blood glucose sampling over one day.

- Carry out a urinalysis and look especially for ketonuria which gives an early warning of instability.

- If the regular three-weekly check-ups show consistently good glycaemic control, then the time interval between visits may be extended.

Treatment of ketoacidosis

This is an uncommon but serious complication of diabetes mellitus. Patients presented exhibiting signs of ketoacidosis should be considered medical emergencies and require immediate medical treatment. Therapy should be directed along the following lines:

Ensure a patent airway

If the patient is collapsed or comatose, an airway must be established using an endotracheal tube if required. ECG monitoring is useful as many cases have significant changes in serum electrolytes which may cause cardiac arrythmias.

Restore fluid balance

Fluid balance should be restored based on calculating the amount of fluid required to correct the dehydration (10ml/kg/1% dehydrated). To this should be added 4ml/kg/vomiting episode and the daily maintenance requirement (40ml/kg/day).

The first 20% should be given in three to four hours and the remainder over the next 20 hours. If fluids are administered too rapidly, cerebral oedema may occur. Hartmann's solution (lactated Ringer's solution) is ideal but where liver function is disturbed, 0.9% saline may be a better choice.

Serum potassium levels are often low in ketoacidosis due to urine losses, osmotic diuresis and excretion of ketones as potassium salts. However, serum potassium levels may initially appear normal or high, due to dehydration and once fluid balance has been restored potassium levels will fall. This will be exacerbated by administration of insulin which drives potassium into cells. Hypokalaemia causes weakness, depression and anorexia, suggesting fluid therapy and insulin administration is failing to work. Potassium should be administered with the Hartmann's solution at rates calculated from the actual serum levels. Similarly, serum phosphate levels may be low, causing haemolysis, profound weakness, rhabdomyolysis and seizures. Correct this by incorporating potassium phosphate into the intravenous fluid administration. It is essential to monitor potassium and phosphate levels after administration.

Restoration of normal blood glucose levels

Remember that ketone production is switched 'on' by glucagon, cortisol, growth hormone and adrenaline and can *only* be switched 'off' by insulin. Neutral insulin should be used in all ketoacidotic patients as it allows rapid onset of action because it can be used intravenously or intramuscularly. It only lasts approximately two hours so good control is also possible. Neutral insulin can be administered in two ways: it can be added to a separate 500ml bag of Hartmann's solution given at a rate which delivers 0.5iu/hour; alternatively, 0.2iu/kg neutral insulin can be given intravenously followed by hourly intramuscular injections of 0.1iu/kg. The use of frequent intravenous boluses of insulin cause marked fluctuations in blood glucose level whereas intramuscular injections help to stabilise blood glucose levels more effectively.

The aim of this treatment is to maintain the blood glucose level between 11 and 16mmol/l. If the blood glucose level falls below 11mmol/l, then 5% dextrose saline should be administered and the hourly intramuscular insulin injections dropped by 10%. If the blood glucose level exceeds 16mmol/l, hourly insulin injections should be increased by 10%.

After the blood glucose level has been maintained at between 11 and 16mmol/l for at least 12 hours and the patient is bright, has stopped vomiting and is hydrated, then 0.5iu/kg lente insulin can be administered subcutaneously every eight to 12 hours while maintaining fluid therapy. Once the patient is able to eat and drink normally, the stabilisation procedure for uncomplicated cases previously described may be started.

Restoration of blood pH

Patients with ketoacidosis are in a state of metabolic acidosis. This means their blood pH is too low and requires to be returned to normal. In most practical situations, this can be done using lactated Ringer's solution. Occasionally, intravenous sodium bicarbonate is required. However, intravenous bicarbonate solutions should not be given to dogs with ketoacidosis unless blood gas analysis is readily available to monitor blood pH.

9 Feline diabetes mellitus

Incidence

Diabetes mellitus occurs most commonly in middle-aged to old cats, with male neutered cats being over-represented. There is no apparent breed predisposition. The incidence of diabetes mellitus in cats is similar to that in dogs.

Aetiology

As previously described, diabetes mellitus occurs due to an absolute or relative insulin deficiency. In contrast to dogs, Type II diabetes, characterised by peripheral tissue resistance to insulin, accounts for a large proportion (at least 30-50%) of cases of feline diabetes. Obesity appears to be an important predisposing factor.

Insulin dependent diabetes mellitus (IDDM) in cats may actually represent a progression of the non insulin dependent form (NIDDM), where prolonged over-stimulation of pancreatic beta-cells leads to eventual exhaustion and an absolute deficiency of insulin. In up to 90% of cases, Type II diabetes in cats is associated with islet amyloidosis. Amylin, which is co-secreted with insulin, becomes deposited around the islet cells. Amyloidosis has been implicated in the progression from NIDDM to IDDM in cats, but it may just be indicative of progressive beta-cell dysfunction.

Transient diabetes mellitus has been observed in cats, whereby treatment with insulin and/or oral hypoglycaemics leads to resolution of the diabetic state. This may be due to chronic hyperglycaemia causing desensitisation and beta-cells becoming refractory to glucose, leading to reduced ability to secrete insulin. It is thought that by re-establishing glycaemic control, beta-cells can recover function and thus remove the need for continued therapy.

Diabetes mellitus in the cat can be secondary to other endocrine and metabolic disorders such as hyperadrenocorticism, hyperthyroidism, acromegaly and pheochromocytoma. Prolonged administration of corticosteroids and megoestrol acetate therapy may also result in overt signs of diabetes mellitus in cats. Inability to stabilise a diabetic cat should prompt the search for an underlying cause.

Clinical signs

Clinical signs of diabetes mellitus are similar to those seen in the dog, with polyphagia, polydipsia, polyuria and weight loss being most common. Occasionally, affected cats will develop a plantigrade stance associated with diabetic neuropathy.

Diagnosis

In cats, the diagnosis of diabetes mellitus can be complicated by the frequent occurrence of stress-induced hyperglycaemia, which can result in serum glucose levels of over 22mmol/l. Diagnosis must, therefore, be based on demonstration of persistent hyperglycaemia and glucosuria. Serum fructosamine, which is formed by the non-enzymatic glycosylation of serum albumin, may be useful in both the diagnosis and management of feline diabetes mellitus as serum levels reflect glucose concentrations over the preceding 2-3 week period. It warrants mentioning that fructosamine can also be elevated with prolonged stress-induced hyperglycaemia.

Treatment

Treatment of feline diabetes mellitus requires a combination of exogenous insulin, oral hypoglycaemic therapy and dietary management. The majority of diabetic cats will require insulin therapy and >75% of cats will require twice daily administration.

Preparations licensed for cats include soluble, lente and protamine zinc (PZI) bovine insulin. Bovine insulin is structurally similar to feline insulin and therefore in theory it should be less antigenic than other types of insulin. Initial therapy should either be with twice daily lente-bovine insulin, at 0.2-0.5iu/kg/dose, or alternatively with PZI-bovine insulin given once daily at 1-3iu/cat. Cats appear to be particularly sensitive to exogenous insulin and therefore the initial dose is much lower than in dogs.

Due to the small doses required it may be necessary to dilute the insulin 1:10 with sterile saline or water to ensure more accurate dosing. It can take up to 3-4 days for the body to equilibrate to a particular dose of insulin. Adjustments to the dose of insulin should be made at this stage on the basis of a blood glucose curve. Incremental increases of no more than 0.5iu/dose should be made.

As with dogs, normalisation of clinical signs is the best indicator of appropriate regulation. Fructosamine and glycosylated haemoglobin may also provide good indications of long-term glycaemic control. After initial stabilisation, it is important to re-evaluate the case on a regular basis.

Dietary management is an important factor in the management of feline diabetes. Avoidance of semi-moist and jelly-coated cat foods which are high in simple sugars and propylene glycol will reduce post-prandial surges in blood glucose. Ad lib feeding of a high fibre diet is ideal, provided calorific intake is monitored closely to avoid weight gain. Weight reduction is important in obese cats and can result in a reduction of insulin requirements. It may occasionally result in resolution of diabetes all together.

Oral hypoglycaemics may be useful in the treatment of feline diabetics. Sulphonylurea drugs, e.g. glipizide, work in part by increasing the production of insulin by remaining pancreatic b-cells and by improving tissue sensitivity to insulin. They are, therefore, dependent on the ability of the pancreas to produce insulin and therefore limited to the treatment of Type II, NIDDM in cats.

The main advantage of using oral hypoglycaemics is that they avoid the necessity to inject the cat with insulin preparations. Response rates are, however, variable. Diabetics that respond to glipizide may subsequently require insulin therapy. Oral hypoglycaemic therapy should be reserved for clinically well, non-ketotic cats whose owners are not prepared to inject them.

- Hill's* Prescription Diet* Feline w/d*: Cats of normal body weight
- Hill's* Prescription Diet* Feline r/d*: Obese cats
- Hill's* Prescription Diet* Feline i/d*: Underweight cats

Figure 11.
Diets which have been specially formulated for the dietary management of feline diabetes mellitus.

10 Complications and instability

Where the insulin requirement exceeds 2iu/kg/day or where blood glucose levels remain high (>14mmol/l), then problems in stabilisation have occurred and further investigation is required.

The vast majority of cases which become unstable occur because of errors in the daily routine and management. Before instigating an expensive and time-consuming investigation, this should be carefully examined as follows:

- The veterinary surgeon and owner should go over the daily routine step by step to ensure it is being carried out correctly.

- Check the insulin is still 'in date' and that it is being stored correctly.

- Check the Keto-diastix or Glucostix are 'in date' and being stored correctly.

- Ensure the animal is not receiving extra food from any source. This can sometimes occur without the owner's knowledge.

- Check the owner's record of events as this may provide useful information.

- If the diabetic is female, ensure she has been spayed. Similarly, check that no insulin antagonistic drugs are being administered. Could the patient have concurrent hyperadrenocorticalism?

Assuming all these factors are in order, the patient should be hospitalised for further investigation of the problem. The first step of such an investigation is to carry out the normal daily routine while monitoring blood glucose levels every two hours for 24 hours. This will provide essential information regarding the underlying cause of the instability. The three most common causes of instability can be summarised as follows:

Insulin induced hyperglycaemia

This is associated with excessive administration of insulin and is sometimes also known as the Somogyi effect. If daily insulin injections are too high, this induces marked hypoglycaemia shortly after injection. This in turn stimulates antagonistic hormones to counter the effect by raising blood glucose levels. This rebound hyperglycaemia can be equally marked and occurs later in the 24-hour period.

With this effect, urine glucose is always positive in the morning, leading to an ever increasing dose of insulin being administered by the owner. The problem is readily identified by serial blood glucose estimations and is easily corrected by reducing the amount of insulin administered each day.

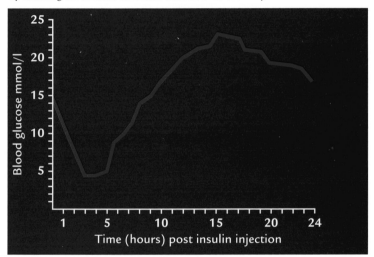

Figure 12.
Blood glucose levels observed with insulin induced hyperglycaemia.
(Courtesy of Schering-Plough Animal Health).

33

Rapid metabolism of insulin

In some dogs, injected insulin is metabolised very rapidly so the response is only maintained for a short period of time (<8 hours in some cases). Therefore, hyperglycaemia develops and glycosuria returns. Monitoring blood glucose levels will reveal a satisfactory initial response to injected insulin followed by a slowly increasing blood glucose level thereafter.

The problem is corrected by using a longer-lasting insulin such as a mixed insulin or protamine zinc insulin or by giving insulin injections twice daily at 12-hour intervals.

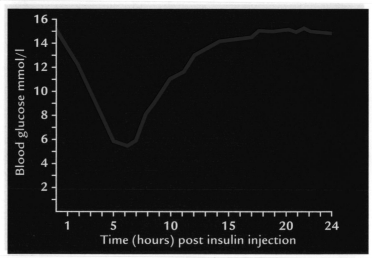

Figure 13.
Rapid metabolism of insulin.
(Courtesy of Schering-Plough Animal Health).

Insulin resistance

Persistent hyperglycaemia and failure to respond to insulin injections strongly suggests insulin resistance. This may be due to concurrent hyperadrenocorticalism, administration of progestagens, glucocorticoids or oestrus. Correction of whichever factor is present restores the response to insulin. Rarely, however, the failure to respond to insulin is due to antibody production against injected insulin, especially if this is a beef insulin. In this situation, changing to a porcine insulin which is structurally identical to canine insulin will correct the problem.

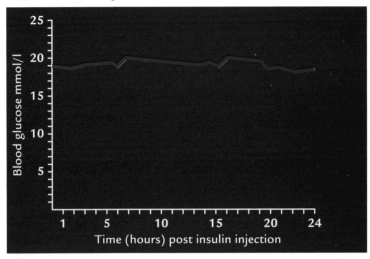

Figure 14.
Insulin insensitivity.
(Courtesy of Schering-Plough Animal Health).

11 Summary

Diabetes mellitus is a relatively common endocrine condition in the dog. It is less common in the cat. Following loss of beta cells from the Islets of Langerhans, there is inadequate production of insulin to control blood glucose levels. Consequently, cells are unable to utilise glucose, hyperglycaemia and glycosuria occur. Initially, patients present with polyuria, polydipsia and polyphagia.

If left untreated, these signs change because the patient tries to use fat and protein as alternative energy sources. The consequence of this change in metabolism is the development of ketoacidosis, resulting in the patient exhibiting anorexia, vomiting, dehydration and depression. A sweet smell of ketones may be detected on the breath and in the urine.

The diagnosis of diabetes rarely presents a problem. It requires the detection of consistent glycosuria in the presence of hyperglycaemia.

Treatment involves the combined use of dietary management and insulin by injection. Initial stabilisation usually takes some two weeks to achieve and if successful will allow the patient to lead a relatively normal life. Where an entire female develops diabetes, it is important she is neutered before her next oestrous cycle, in order to prevent a relapse.

A sudden loss of stability is not common as long as the owner maintains the strict daily regime. Occasionally, complications associated with insulin resistance, rapid metabolism of insulin and rebound hyperglycaemia may occur, requiring further investigation and alteration in case management.

Appendix 1

Owner's Guide to the Treatment of Diabetes Mellitus

This is an example of the type of document which may be given to owners in order to help them understand the day to day management of their pet with diabetes mellitus. It will require modification for use in patients where blood glucose is used to assess stability and for those receiving twice daily insulin injections. It is intended to offer the reader a guide to the information which may be given to owners.

This document describes the home care for:

Name   Breed
_____

Age   Sex
_____

Three procedures must be carried out each day:

- Maintenance of a strict dietary regime.
- Collection of a urine sample, measurement of the glucose level and calculation of the insulin dose.
- Injecting insulin.

Details of the procedures

Diet

The prescribed diet must be given to the exclusion of all other foods. This will ensure your pet's daily intake of sugar is kept constant. The daily diet should consist of:

_____

_____

_____

This daily diet should be fed as two meals. A quarter of the ration should be given in the morning and the remaining three-quarters in the afternoon.

Give the morning meal at: _____

Give the afternoon meal at: _____

ALWAYS ensure there is a supply of fresh water available.

NEVER feed extra meals or tit-bits as this will cause your pet to become unstable.

Urine glucose measurement

The purpose of urine testing is to ensure that the correct amount of insulin is given each day. The level of glucose in the urine should be maintained at 1/10 to 1/4 percent (14 to 28mmol/l).

The urine sample should be collected in a clean container at the same time each day and tested for glucose according to the instructions enclosed with the reagent strips.

This will allow you to determine the daily insulin requirement of your pet. In general, the insulin dose required may be determined using the Table below. (See Table on page 24). If the other reagent strip (for ketones) changes colour, telephone your veterinary surgeon for advice.

Administration of insulin

Inject _____ units of insulin at _____ am/pm each day.

Remove the insulin from the fridge and gently rock the bottle to mix the contents. Do NOT shake the bottle as this will damage the insulin. Draw the required amount of insulin into a disposable insulin syringe and check your figure before injecting your pet. Return the insulin to the fridge.

Insulin should be injected under the skin and NOT into a vein or a muscle. Use the loose skin along your pet's back as the injection site.

Insert the needle through the skin, draw back on the syringe to ensure the needle has not entered a vein, and if no blood enters the syringe, inject the insulin.

Problems

If your pet does not eat its morning meal, DO NOT inject the insulin. This will cause no harm and will prevent insulin over-dosage and hypoglycaemia from occurring.

If for any reason you have problems injecting the insulin and are not sure how much has been injected, do NOT repeat or 'top up' the insulin dose. Make a note of the problem and administer the correct dose of insulin at the next injection time.

Please keep a detailed record of the date, urine glucose level, insulin dose given and amounts fed each day. This will help if any problems arise with stabilisation and will assist your veterinary surgeon to assess progress at each revisit.

39

Signs of insulin over-dosage

If your pet receives too much insulin, the effect is most likely to be observed about eight hours after injection. Signs can, however, occur earlier or later than this in individuals. The first signs of hypoglycaemia caused by over-dosage of insulin include: muscle tremor, staggering or unsteady limb movements. This will be followed rapidly by collapse and unconsciousness. Treat these signs immediately by giving a level dessertspoonful of glucose or sugar in a little water, orally. If your pet becomes unconscious or you are not sure what to do, do not administer oral glucose but take your pet immediately to your veterinary surgeon.

Appendix 2

Insulinoma

Introduction

Unlike diabetes mellitus, insulinoma is a rare hormonal condition of the dog and cat. Insulinoma is a function tumour of the beta cells of the pancreas which results in secretion of excess insulin. These tumours tend to be very small and difficult to detect even when examining the pancreas at surgery or at post mortem. The degree of malignancy varies but spread to the local lymph nodes, liver and lung does occur. High insulin levels associated with insulinoma result in profound hypoglycaemia and failure of glucose homeostasis.

Incidence

Although insulinoma may occur in any breed of dog, they appear most frequently in the larger breeds such as the German Shepherd, Irish Setter, Airedale, Boxer and Golden Retriever. There is no sex predisposition but most cases occur in dogs between eight and 12 years of age. Insulinoma has been documented in the Siamese cat.

Clinical signs

It is essential that blood glucose levels are maintained within very narrow limits because the central nervous system is dependent on correct levels of blood glucose to function. Consequently, beta cell tumours result in hyperinsulinism and profound hypoglycaemia which results in patients exhibiting central nervous symptoms.

Clinical signs exhibited vary from case to case and this may be due to the degree of hypoglycaemia present and the level of antagonistic hormone activity (cortisol, glucagon, growth hormone). Typically, dogs exhibit muscle weakness, exercise intolerance, behavioural changes, unsteadiness on their limbs (ataxia) followed by collapse and seizures. Many patients are polyphagic and may be thin or obese. The presence of clinical signs may be episodic and most frequently occur during fasting and improve following feeding.

Diagnosis

The clinical history will strongly suggest insulinoma; however, there are other conditions which can cause episodic weakness and collapse (Figure 15).

Radiographs are of little value as tumours are very small in size. Ultrasound examination of the pancreas may detect small masses supportive of insulinoma. Ideally, Whipple's Triad should be demonstrated. This requires demonstration of:

- The presence of clinical signs following a period of fasting.

- Blood glucose to be <2mmol/l during the presence of clinical signs.

- Reversal of clinical signs following administration of glucose.

Most often dogs will be admitted for serial blood glucose measurement over 24 hours. This will detect a period of hypoglycaemia. To obtain a definitive diagnosis it is essential to demonstrate high circulating insulin levels at the same time as profound hypoglycaemia. This indicates an inappropriate response to low blood glucose levels.

Epilepsy

Cardiac insufficiency - Bradydysrhythmias of the Boxer

Respiratory disease - failure to oxygenate

Severe anaemia

Central nervous tumours

Encephalitis

Hypoadrenocorticism

Azotaemia

Hepatoencephalopathy

Figure 15.
Other conditions which may cause episodic collapse in the dog.

Treatment

The most effective long-term treatment for insulinoma is surgical removal of the tumour masses from the pancreas and local lymph nodes. Patients should be prepared for surgery by instigating a feeding programme using small, frequent meals to reduce the periods of hypoglycaemia. In addition, glucocorticoids at 0.5mg/kg may be provided to increase the blood glucose levels. Prior to and during surgery, an intravenous infusion of glucose saline should be administered.

Surgery can prove difficult and it is not always successful because of the difficulty in finding the small size of islet cell tumours. In addition, if spread to other tissues has occurred, surgery will not resolve the clinical signs. Rough handling of the pancreas during surgery may result in pancreatitis.

Following surgery several outcomes are possible:

- The patient may continue to have episodes of hypoglycaemia, indicating failure to remove all tumour cells.

- The patient may develop transient diabetes mellitus due to atrophy of remaining normal beta cells.

- The patient may go into remission and remain normoglycaemic.

- The patient may develop pancreatitis.

A remission of clinical signs can be expected in the majority of cases, although clinical signs frequently recur within 12 to 18 months, due to proliferation of undetected tumour cells. The long-term prognosis must, therefore, always remain guarded, although quality of life is generally good during the period of remission.

Where the patient eventually relapses or where the owner declines surgery, medical management can be attempted. This involves feeding small, frequent meals each day together with administration of low doses of glucocorticoids.

Appendix 3

Exocrine pancreatic insufficiency (EPI)

Canine

Aetiology

The majority of the pancreas is composed of exocrine tissue which produces digestive enzymes, including trypsin, amylase and lipase. These enzymes are transported from the pancreas via the pancreatic ducts to the duodenum where they digest food.

Exocrine pancreatic insufficiency (EPI) occurs when there is inadequate enzyme production and subsequent failure of the digestive process. There is a large functional reserve of exocrine tissue so digestive failure only occurs when more than 90% of the exocrine tissue is lost. No loss of endocrine function occurs in EPI, so concurrent diabetes mellitus is very rare in dogs.

Exocrine pancreatic insufficiency can occur in the cat but this is a very rare condition compared with dogs. The loss of exocrine tissue can occur in several ways. In adult dogs EPI is associated with destruction of exocrine tissue following repeated episodes of pancreatitis. However, EPI is much more common in young adult dogs between one and two years of age. In this group there is hypoplasia of the exocrine tissue resulting in EPI, which may be heritable in the German Shepherd dog.

In general, EPI is most common in young dogs of the larger breeds, especially the German Shepherd, Golden Retriever, Rough Collie and Irish Setter.

Clinical signs

Classically, dogs with EPI are said to be 'starving in the presence of plenty'. In spite of ingesting an adequate diet, they are unable to digest the nutrients which subsequently appear in the faeces. Consequently, dogs with EPI exhibit signs associated with maldigestion.

43

In particular, they exhibit a ravenous appetite (polyphagia), lose significant amounts of body weight (>30%), produce large volumes of chronic foul smelling diarrhoea and may practice coprophagia (eating their own faeces). In spite of the significant weight loss associated with EPI, dogs frequently remain bright and active. Secondary problems, however, may develop, including poor skin and coat condition, increased susceptibility to infection and failure to show signs of oestrus.

Diagnosis

A tentative diagnosis of EPI can be made from the clinical signs and examination of the faeces for the presence of undigested fat and starch. A definitive diagnosis requires the collection of a fasted serum sample to measure trypsinogen-like immunoreactivity (TLI test). In normal dogs, significant amounts of trypsinogen 'leak' from the pancreas into the circulation; in dogs with EPI, very little trypsinogen 'leaks' into the circulation, resulting in very low TLI values (<2.5ug/l).

Treatment

The treatment of EPI is both expensive and time-consuming for the owner. For this reason it is important for the veterinary surgeon to discuss the proposed treatment regime with the owner. The aims of treating dogs with EPI should be to reverse the principal clinical signs in the following chronological order:

- Correct the chronic diarrhoea.

- Restore the dog's body weight.

- Eliminate the ravenous appetite.

The restoration of normal faecal character can be achieved by feeding a low fat veterinary diet together with replacement enzyme supplement in two meals daily. This diet must be fed to the exclusion of all other foods, which can be very difficult because of the dog's ravenous appetite. The diet should initially be fed according to the dog's present body weight, in order to establish the passage of normal faeces. This usually occurs within 48 to 72 hours of starting the new regime.

After normal faeces have been consistently produced, the diet can be slowly increased until weight gain is achieved. Restoration of normal body weight may take two to three months to achieve. Attempts to achieve this in a shorter period of time, by rapidly increasing the amount fed each day, will result in recurrence of the chronic diarrhoea.

Only after the dog's body weight has been restored to normal will the ravenous appetite decline. At this time, the amount of low fat veterinary diet and replacement enzyme can usually be reduced to a level which will maintain the dog's normal body weight. This will significantly reduce the long-term cost of treatment. Approximately 75% of dogs with EPI will respond successfully to this treatment regime.

Feline

Exocrine pancreatic insufficiency is extremely rare in the cat. The hereditary and congenital forms seen in the dog do not occur in the cat. Most cases of feline EPI are associated with chronic pancreatitis and long-term destruction of exocrine tissue. Therefore, cats more commonly develop EPI in middle or old age.

Clinical signs of feline EPI are similar to those observed in the dog, with weight loss, ravenous appetite and chronic diarrhoea. It is very important to consider other causes of these signs such as inflammatory bowel disease, which is much more common than EPI. A diagnosis of EPI requires measurement of specific feline TLI. At present this can only be measured by a laboratory at Texas A&M University. The canine TLI should not be used.

Treatment of feline EPI requires the use of a highly digestible diet together with enzyme replacer. Reducing the level of fat in the diet is not as important in cats as it is in dogs. In fact, the cat relies on fat as an energy source to a much greater degree than carbohydrates, which are less well tolerated in the species. Protocols for the use of diet and enzyme supplements are similar to those described for the dog.

45

Glossary

Alopecia:	Hair loss.
ADH:	Antidiuretic hormone which acts on kidney collecting ducts to conserve water
Auto-immune:	A condition characterised by an immune response by the animal against its own body tissues.
Azotaemia:	An abnormal increase in the serum concentrations of urea and creatinine together with other waste products.
Cacinosis cutis:	Deposition of calcium in the skin.
Cystitis:	Inflammation of the urinary bladder.
DNA:	Deoxyribonucleic acid found within the nucleus of cells where genetic material is stored.
Disaccharide:	Two simple sugars joined together, for example sucrose and lactose.
ECG:	Electrocardiograph.
Endocrine:	An endocrine gland is one which secretes a hormone directly into the circulation.
Gluconeogenesis:	The formation of glucose from non carbohydrate sources such as from amino acid.
Glycogenolysis:	The breakdown of glycogen in the liver or muscle releasing glucose.
Hepatomegaly:	An increase in the size of the liver.
Hepatotoxin:	A chemical or other agent which damages the liver.
Hormone:	A chemical messenger produced by an endocrine gland which enters the circulation and targets a distant organ.
Hyperglycaemia:	A greater than normal increase in blood glucose level.
HAC:	Hyperadrenocorticalism or Cushing's disease. There is a pathological increase in adrenal cortex function leading to excessive amounts of circulating cortisol.
Hypoglycaemia:	A reduction from normal in the blood glucose level.

Isothenuria: Refers to urine of the same concentration as plasma
                            and which has not been subject to concentration.
                            SG = 1.009 to 1.012

Ketoacidosis: An accumulation of ketones in the circulation and the
                            presence of metabolic acidosis.

Leucocytosis: An increase from normal in the number of circulating
                            white blood cells.

Metabolic acidosis: A condition which results in an increase in the acidity
                            of body; most frequently associated with the
                            production of metabolic acids and/or loss of
                            bicarbonate.

Metabolism: All the physical and chemical processes by which the
                            body is maintained and energy formed for work to be
                            carried out.

Monosaccharide: A simple sugar such as glucose.

Myopathy: Any disease of the skeletal muscle.

Neuropathy: Any disease of the central or peripheral nerves.

Pancreatitis: Inflammation of the pancreas.

Pathognomonic: Indicative of a particular disease.

Polydipsia: An increase in thirst above normal,
                            excessive water intake.

Polysaccharide: A complex sugar such as starch which is composed of
                            many thousands of glucose units joined together.

Polyuria: An abnormal increase in urine production and output.

Renal medullary   Loss of sodium, chloride and urea from the renal
washout: medulla as a result of polyuria. There is inability to
                            concentrate the urine.

Urinalysis: Analysis of a urine sample.

PWDT: The partial water deprivation test used to determine if
                            an animal can concentrate its urine.

Daily Record Sheet

Date	Urine glucose	Urine Ketones	Insulin Dose		Meals First		Second		Notes
			Time	Amt	Time	Amt	Time	Amt	